MUCUNA PRURIENS FOR BEGINNERS

Harnessing Mucuna Pruriens , A Comprehensive Guide To Unlocking The Nature's Answer To Vitality Benefits, And Holistic Wellness

Georgette Lockett

© [2023] [Georgette Lockett]

DISCLAIMER

The author of this book is not affiliated, associated, endorsed, sponsored, or approved by any company or individual. The views and opinions expressed in this book are solely those of the author and do not necessarily reflect the official policy or position of any entity.

The author hereby disclaims any relationship, collaboration, or partnership with any company or individual mentioned in this book. Any references to products, services, or individuals are provided for informational purposes only and should not be construed as an endorsement or recommendation.

Readers are advised to exercise their own judgment and discretion when applying the information provided in this book. The author shall not be held responsible for any actions taken by readers based on the content of this book.

This book is intended for general informational purposes only, and the author makes no representations or warranties of any kind, express or implied, about the completeness, accuracy, reliability, suitability, or availability of the information contained herein. Any reliance on the information in this book is at the reader's own risk.

The author reserves the right to update, change, or modify any information in this book without notice. It is the responsibility of the reader to verify any information before taking any actions based on the content of this book.

By reading this book, the reader acknowledges and agrees to the terms of this disclaimer.

Table of Contents

INTRODUCTION

Mucuna Pruriens, often known as velvet bean or cowhage, is a leguminous plant with complex qualities and medicinal potential that has been used for generations. This tropical legume has a long history, strongly entwined with numerous civilizations for its varied purposes in traditional medicine. Mucuna Pruriens, revered for its wide range of advantages, continues to fascinate interest in current scientific research and alternative health practices.

Overview Of Mucuna Pruriens

Mucuna pruriens is a climbing plant that is endemic to tropical places such as Africa, India, and the Caribbean. Its unique look, with long green pods coated with bristles, contains therapeutic seeds.

Historical Roots: The plant has a long history in traditional medicine, most notably in Ayurveda,

Traditional Chinese Medicine (TCM), and African herbal therapies. Its historical use includes treating a variety of diseases such as nervous system problems, and male infertility, and as an antidote for snakebites.

Active Compounds: L-DOPA (L-3,4-dihydroxyphenylalanine) is a precursor of dopamine, which is required for neurotransmitter production. Mucuna Pruriens includes alkaloids, flavonoids, saponins, and other bioactive substances in addition to L-DOPA, which contribute to its medicinal benefits.

Importance And Historical Uses

Traditional Therapeutic Applications: Various civilizations have used Mucuna Pruriens for its therapeutic benefits throughout history. It is known as Kapikachhu in Ayurveda and is said to promote energy, reproductive health, and neurological well-being. TCM incorporates it to improve kidney function and manage yang deficient concerns.

The herb has cultural significance and is often utilized in rituals and celebrations among indigenous tribes. Its seeds, leaves, and roots were prized for their purported medicinal powers and spiritual importance.

Significance In Modern Medicine And Research

Scientific Interest: Because of its possible medicinal uses, Mucuna Pruriens has recently sparked a boom in scientific interest. Researchers are looking into its neuroprotective, antioxidant, and anti-inflammatory characteristics to see whether it might help with ailments including Parkinson's disease, mood problems, and infertility.

Pharmacological Investigation: The presence of L-DOPA in Mucuna Pruriens has sparked interest due to its potential significance in Parkinson's disease therapy as a natural alternative to synthetic dopamine. Studies are being conducted to investigate its bioavailability, dosing effectiveness, and comparative advantages over traditional drugs.

Mucuna Pruriens pills have acquired appeal in the domain of holistic health among persons seeking natural therapies to boost mood, cognitive function, and general well-being.

The Introduction to Mucuna Pruriens establishes the groundwork for a thorough examination of its historical relevance, multiple uses in traditional medicine, and increasing prominence in current scientific research and alternative health practices.

CHAPTER 1

Botanical Profile Of Mucuna Pruriens

Mucuna pruriens, often known as velvet bean or cowhage, is a leguminous plant with several uses in traditional medicine and current science. Let's take a closer look at its botanical profile:

Taxonomy And Classification

Mucuna pruriens is a member of the Fabaceae family, specifically the subfamily Faboideae. In this family, it belongs to the genus Mucuna. Mucuna pruriens (L.) DC is the scientific name for it. The word "pruriens" is derived from the Latin verb "prurio," which means "to itch," and refers to the skin irritation produced by the plant's bristles upon contact.

Morphological Characteristics

Mucuna pruriens is a climbing shrub with thin, twining stems that may grow to be several meters long. Its growth pattern allows it to climb and entangle with other plants.

- **Leaves:** The trifoliate, alternating leaves have a velvety touch. Each leaf has three leaflets that are oblong to lanceolate in form and have pointy points.

- **Flowers:** The plant has striking purple or lavender flowers that are grouped in racemes. These pendulous flower clusters include both male and female reproductive organs.

- **Fruits and Seeds:** The plant grows pods (legumes) with thick, bristly hairs. The seeds, which are generally dark brown and irregular in form, are contained inside these pods. Because of its therapeutic powers, the seeds are the most sought-after portion.

Habitat And Geographical Distribution

Mucuna pruriens is native to tropical and subtropical climates, primarily in Africa, Asia, and the Caribbean. It may be found in a wide range of environments, including woods, grasslands, and disturbed regions. It grows well in warm, humid climates with well-drained soil.

Because of the plant's versatility, it has naturalized in many areas outside of its original habitat, increasing its availability for both traditional and modern purposes.

Understanding Mucuna prurient botanical features offers the groundwork for understanding its many uses in traditional medicine, agriculture, and continuing scientific research.

CHAPTER 2

Chemical Composition

Mucuna pruriens, popularly known as velvet bean or cowhage, is a tropical leguminous plant. Because of its complex chemical content, their seeds have been used in traditional medicine for generations. Its pharmacological activities are aided by several active substances.

Active Compounds And Their Properties

1. **L-DOPA (Levodopa):** L-DOPA, a precursor to the neurotransmitters dopamine, norepinephrine, and epinephrine, is the star of Mucuna pruriens. L-DOPA's neuroprotective effects make it an important therapeutic component in the treatment of neurological diseases such as Parkinson's disease.

2. **Alkaloids:** Mucunine, mucunadine, and other alkaloids are found in the plant.

While their specific function is unknown, these alkaloids are expected to contribute to the plant's overall pharmacological action.

3. Tryptamines: Tryptamine derivatives such as serotonin and 5-hydroxytryptamine have been discovered in trace levels. These chemicals are essential for mood modulation and nervous system function.

4. Proteins and Amino Acids: Mucuna seeds contain proteins that include all necessary amino acids, adding to their nutritional value.

5. Flavonoids and Phenolic Compounds: These antioxidants have been shown to have anti-inflammatory and neuroprotective properties.

L-Dopa Content And Its Significance

Because of its involvement in dopamine production, L-DOPA is of special relevance. Parkinson's disease is related to dopamine insufficiency, and L-DOPA supplementation has been a cornerstone in its therapy. Mucuna prurience L-DOPA content, in a natural matrix among other bioactive substances, is thought to provide tolerance and efficacy benefits than synthetic L-DOPA.

Mucuna pruriens contains L-DOPA, which has prompted interest in its possible application not just in Parkinson's disease but also in other disorders involving dopamine imbalance or insufficiency.

Other Bioactive Components

Mucuna pruriens includes a variety of bioactive ingredients, including polysaccharides, saponins, phytosterols, and fatty acids, which contribute to its pharmacological activities.

These substances interact synergistically, and their combined activity may have a more comprehensive therapeutic impact than individual components, while more study is required to understand their specific processes and possible health benefits.

The complex chemical makeup of Mucuna pruriens underpins its traditional and modern medical uses, making it a target for researchers looking for innovative treatment alternatives and formulations.

CHAPTER 3
Traditional Uses

Mucuna Pruriens, often known as velvet bean or cowhage, plays an important role in traditional medicine systems across the globe, with a long history of ethnobotanical applications in many cultures. Its origins may be traced back to ancient civilizations when it was valued for its medical benefits and distinct traits.

Ethnobotanical History

Mucuna pruriens has a lengthy history that is strongly ingrained in traditional medicinal techniques. It has been grown and used for ages in many regions of the globe. Various indigenous groups in Africa, Asia, and South America have traditionally used various sections of the Mucuna Pruriens plant for medicinal reasons.

Traditional Medicinal Uses Across Cultures

Ayurveda:

Mucuna pruriens has been valued as an essential plant in Ayurveda, the ancient Indian school of medicine, for its possible health benefits. It is classed as an adaptogen, and it is said to increase energy and stamina. Ayurvedic practitioners have employed various components of the plant, particularly the seeds, to treat a variety of health issues.

TCM (Traditional Chinese Medicine):

Mucuna Pruriens is renowned in TCM for its function in kidney tonification and is said to be useful for stimulating libido, improving mood, and promoting general vitality. It is often employed in formulae aimed at replenishing Jing (life essence) and treating kidney-related ailments.

Mucuna pruriens has been used for a variety of reasons by communities in Africa and South America for centuries. The seeds, in particular, have been utilized to treat snakebites, skin diseases, and nervous system issues. It's also used as an anthelmintic to get rid of parasitic worms.

Folklore And Cultural Significance

Mucuna pruriens has long had symbolic and cultural value in several locations, apart from its therapeutic purpose. It is considered auspicious in certain societies and is utilized in rites or festivities. Its distinct look and powerful capabilities have made it a topic of folklore and cultural legends in many countries, often signifying fertility, vigor, or protection against harmful forces.

In conclusion, Mucuna Pruriens has historical and cultural relevance in a variety of civilizations and traditional therapeutic techniques. Its many uses in various cultures not only demonstrate its versatility but also signal its potential utility in contemporary medicine, piquing scientific curiosity and prompting continuous study into its pharmacological qualities.

CHAPTER 4

Pharmacological Properties

Neuroprotective Effects

Mucuna Pruriens is well-known for its neuroprotective properties. L-DOPA, a precursor to dopamine, is found in the seeds and is essential for brain processes. Dopamine aids in the regulation of mood, locomotion, and emotional reactions. L-DOPA from Mucuna Pruriens has been demonstrated in studies to have neuroprotective properties, possibly benefiting illnesses such as Parkinson's disease. Compounds in the plant may protect neurons from oxidative stress, lowering the incidence of neurodegenerative illnesses.

Antioxidant Properties

Because of the presence of different bioactive substances such as flavonoids, phenolic acids, and alkaloids, the plant has powerful antioxidant properties. These components help the body scavenge damaging free radicals, reducing oxidative damage to cells and tissues. The antioxidant activity of Mucuna Pruriens adds to its general health advantages, which include anti-aging effects and protection against chronic illnesses.

Antidiabetic Potential

Mucuna pruriens has shown encouraging results in the treatment of diabetes. According to some studies, its hypoglycemic qualities may help manage blood sugar levels. Compounds present in the seeds, including L-DOPA and some flavonoids, may help with insulin release and glucose metabolism. It may also protect against diabetic problems due to its antioxidant and anti-inflammatory properties.

Antimicrobial Properties

Several researches have revealed Mucuna Pruriens' antibacterial capabilities. Extracts from various sections of the plant have antibacterial, antifungal, and antiviral properties against a variety of diseases. These features imply that they might be used to treat microbial infections, although further study is required to understand precise pathways and therapeutic consequences.

With its diverse pharmacological characteristics, Mucuna Pruriens offers great potential in contemporary medicine. Its neuroprotective qualities, antioxidant capacity, anti-diabetic characteristics, and antibacterial activity have piqued the interest of scientists. While these results are encouraging, further thorough clinical trials are needed to completely evaluate and understand the processes behind these outcomes. Mucuna Pruriens' traditional applications throughout cultures highlight its historical significance and possible usefulness in modern healthcare treatments.

CHAPTER 5

Therapeutic Applications

Mucuna pruriens, popularly known as velvet bean, has gotten a lot of interest for its many medicinal uses. Let us now look at Chapter 5, with an emphasis on its therapeutic benefits:

Parkinson's Disease Management

Mucuna pruriens is noteworthy for its ability to treat Parkinson's disease. It is rich in L-DOPA, a precursor to dopamine, which is low in Parkinson's patients. Mucuna pruriens L-DOPA supplementation has shown encouraging benefits in relieving motor symptoms and overall quality of life in Parkinson's patients. Furthermore, the presence of additional substances in the plant may supplement the benefits of L-DOPA, thereby lowering the adverse effects associated with synthetic L-DOPA treatments.

Mental Health Benefits

Mucuna pruriens's chemical makeup leads to its mental health advantages. Aside from its effect on Parkinson's, its L-DOPA content promotes brain health by possibly increasing dopamine levels, which may improve mood control, cognition, and general mental well-being. Some studies show that its neuroprotective characteristics may aid in the management of stress, anxiety, and depression, while more study is required to completely understand these effects.

Sexual Health And Fertility

Mucuna pruriens has been utilized in different traditional medical traditions to treat sexual health concerns and infertility. Its aphrodisiac potential is related to its effect on dopamine levels, which may increase libido and sexual desire. Furthermore, Mucuna pruriens may improve male fertility by enhancing sperm quality, motility, and count.

has prompted research into its usage in resolving male reproductive health difficulties.

Other Potential Therapeutic Uses

Aside from the aforementioned applications, the current study has looked at Mucuna pruriens' potential medicinal uses. These are some examples:

• **Antioxidant and anti-inflammatory properties:** Antioxidant substances found in plants, including flavonoids and alkaloids, can battle oxidative stress and inflammation, both of which are linked to a variety of disorders.

• **Neuroprotective Effects:** Mucuna pruriens may give neuroprotective effects against neurodegenerative illnesses such as Alzheimer's disease owing to its potential to increase dopamine levels and antioxidant qualities.

• **Diabetes Management:** Some study suggests that Mucuna pruriens may help manage diabetes by adjusting blood sugar levels and enhancing insulin sensitivity, but further research is required to confirm its usefulness and safety.

Understanding Mucuna's prurient therapeutic potential across several areas emphasizes its importance in current healthcare. However, further clinical studies and research are required to test its effectiveness, define ideal doses, and identify any adverse effects to ensure its safe and successful use in a variety of therapeutic applications.

CHAPTER 6

Clinical Studies And Research

Mucuna Pruriens, often known as velvet bean, has piqued the curiosity of scientists owing to its several potential health advantages. In this chapter, we'll look at clinical trials and research related to this fascinating plant.

Overview Of Clinical Trials

Clinical studies are critical for evaluating Mucuna Pruriens' safety, effectiveness, and prospective uses in a variety of medical disorders. Several studies have been done throughout the years to better understand its pharmacological characteristics and therapeutic potential. These trials usually consist of many stages:

1. Phase I trials are designed to assess safety, determine appropriate doses, and evaluate side effects in a small sample of healthy volunteers.

2. Phase II trials include a bigger sample size and are designed to evaluate the effectiveness of Mucuna Pruriens in treating particular ailments. Participants in these studies are often diagnosed with Parkinson's disease, mental health issues, sexual dysfunction, and other conditions.

3. Phase III trials are large-scale investigations that are carried out to further analyze effectiveness, monitor side effects, and compare the therapy to established standards or placebos.

Efficacy And Safety Assessments

Parkinson's Disease Care:

Mucuna pruriens has received interest for its possible use in the treatment of Parkinson's disease. L-DOPA, a precursor to dopamine, a neurotransmitter essential for motor function, is found in the plant. According to research, the natural L-DOPA found in Mucuna Pruriens may be superior to synthetic L-DOPA in terms of adverse effects and enhanced motor control. Clinical studies have shown excellent findings, proving its usefulness in treating Parkinson's disease symptoms.

Mental Health Advantages:

Mucuna pruriens has been studied for its effect on mental health disorders such as depression, anxiety, and stress. Some studies show that it can improve mood, reduce stress, and improve general mental well-being, potentially owing to its dopaminergic and antioxidant qualities. However, further rigorous clinical studies are required to confirm these results.

Fertility and Sexual Health:

Mucuna pruriens has traditionally been used in Ayurvedic medicine to treat male sexual dysfunction and infertility. Some studies have shown that it may boost libido, improve sperm quality, and perhaps increase testosterone levels.

More rigorous clinical studies, however, are necessary to corroborate these results and establish the mechanism of action.

Other Potential Therapeutic Applications

Aside from the aforementioned domains, the continuing study is looking at Mucuna Pruriens' possible medicinal uses. This includes its involvement in:

• **Neurological Disorders:** In addition to Parkinson's disease, research is being conducted to investigate its potential in the treatment of other neurological disorders.

• **Antioxidant and Anti-inflammatory characteristics:** According to research, its antioxidant and anti-inflammatory characteristics may have wider implications in the treatment of many disorders.

- **Metabolic Health:** Some research suggests that it may be useful in managing blood sugar levels and boosting metabolic health indicators.

Future Research Directions

Mucuna Pruriens's research is extensive and ever-changing. Future research is expected to dive further into:

- **Extract Standardization:** Creating standardized extracts and formulations for improved consistency and effectiveness.

- **Long-term Safety and effectiveness:** Long-term studies to investigate long-term safety and effectiveness in a variety of groups.

- **Mechanistic Understanding:** Deciphering the specific processes behind its therapeutic actions to improve targeted therapies.

In conclusion, while existing research provides promising insights into Mucuna Pruriens' potential therapeutic applications, well-designed clinical trials and in-depth research are required to validate its efficacy, safety, and diverse applications in medicine and human health.

CHAPTER 7

Cultivation And Harvesting

Mucuna Pruriens, often known as velvet bean, is a legume with therapeutic effects. To guarantee maximum development and effectiveness in medicinal applications, this plant must be grown and harvested using precise processes.

Cultivation Techniques

1. Soil and Climate: Mucuna Pruriens grows best in warm, humid regions. It thrives on well-drained, sandy loam soils with pH levels ranging from slightly acidic to neutral (pH 6.0-7.0). It cannot tolerate cold and needs a minimum temperature of roughly 20°C (68°F) to grow.

2. Propagation: Seeds are commonly used to propagate the plant. Scarification (nicking or scraping the seed coat) may be performed on the seeds before planting to improve germination.

Seeds are often put straight into the soil or in containers, with around 2 meters between rows.

3. Watering & Irrigation: An adequate water supply is critical, particularly during the early phases of development. Excessive moisture, on the other hand, may result in fungal illnesses. Watering measures that are balanced and minimize waterlogging are critical.

4. Fertilization: Incorporating organic matter into the soil before planting aids in the provision of necessary nutrients. Balanced fertilizing throughout the growth phases promotes healthy plant development.

5. Weed and pest control: During the early phases of development, regular weeding is required. Organic pest management measures are suggested to retain the therapeutic qualities of the plant.

Ideal Growing Conditions

- **Temperature:** Mucuna Pruriens grows in tropical and subtropical settings with consistently warm temperatures.

- **Sunshine:** For a large portion of the day, the plant enjoys full sunshine exposure.

- **Humidity:** It thrives in high humidity, although excellent air movement is required to avoid fungal illnesses.

Harvesting And Processing Methods

- **Harvesting Period:** Harvesting occurs when the pods become brown or black and are completely grown. To avoid mold formation, the pods should be dried before harvesting.

- **Harvesting Methods:** Pods are gathered manually by cutting the plant at ground level. Avoiding direct touch with the plant's stinging hairs found on pods and leaves requires caution.

• **Processing:** The pods are dried in a well-ventilated place after harvesting. When the pods are dry, they are threshed to remove the seeds from the pods. The seeds are then ground or extracted to create a variety of formulations such as capsules, tinctures, or extracts.

Following these growing procedures and perfect circumstances provides a robust output of Mucuna Pruriens while retaining its medicinal ingredients. Furthermore, sustainable agricultural techniques are critical for preserving the natural balance and ensuring the survival of this therapeutic plant species.

CHAPTER 8

Formulations And Dosage

Mucuna pruriens, often known as velvet bean or cowhage, is a tropical legume extensively recognized in traditional medicine for its medicinal potential and numerous uses. As we go through Chapter 8, which focuses on formulations and dosage, it becomes clear that the many accessible forms, suggested doses, and administration techniques all play an important part in efficiently using its advantages.

Different Forms Available (Powder, Extract, Supplements)

1. Mucuna pruriens powder is obtained from the dried seeds of the plant and is widely accessible. This form is adaptable, since it may be combined with drinks, meals, or encapsulated for ingestion.

2. Extracts: Extracts are concentrated versions of the plant's active ingredients. They come in a variety of concentrations and are often utilized in supplements or therapeutic formulations.

3. Mucuna pruriens supplements are available in a variety of formulations that combine the plant extract with additional substances to improve bioavailability or augment its benefits.

Recommended Dosages

Dosages might vary depending on variables such as the individual's health, age, and the kind of Mucuna pruriens utilized. Specific doses may change across research and products. Here are some broad principles, however:

• **Powder:** A normal mucuna pruriens powder dose ranges from 500mg to 1000mg used once or twice a day. The concentration of active chemicals in the powder may influence this.

- **Extracts:** Because extracts are more concentrated, they may need lesser dosages. Depending on the concentration, dosages might vary from 100mg to 500mg.

- **Supplements:** Supplement dosages are often supplied by the manufacturer and should be followed as directed on the product label. It is best to get individualized dose advice from a healthcare expert.

Administration Methods

- **Oral Ingestion:** This is the most usual form of administration. Powder or capsules may be taken orally or added to food or drinks.

- **Sublingual:** For faster absorption into the circulation, certain preparations may recommend sublingual administration (putting the material beneath the tongue).

- **Topical Application:** While less prevalent, mucuna pruriens extracts have been used topically in select situations, notably in traditional medicine for problems such as skin irritation.

Important Considerations

- **Consultation:** It is critical to see a healthcare practitioner before beginning any supplement plan, particularly if you have pre-existing health concerns or are taking other drugs.

- **Quality and acquisition:** Because product quality varies, it is best to acquire supplements from recognized manufacturers or approved sources to guarantee effectiveness and safety.

- **Adherence to Recommendations:** To minimize possible detrimental effects associated with excessive ingestion, always stick to prescribed doses.

Mucuna pruriens, in all of its forms, provides a wide range of health advantages. Its effectiveness and usefulness, however, are dependent on optimal formulation, dose, and administration. Understanding these elements is critical for increasing therapeutic potential while limiting dangers. Always seek the opinion of a healthcare expert while using mucuna pruriens for health and wellness reasons.

CHAPTER 9

Side Effects And Precautions

Potential Adverse Effects

1. Nausea and Digestive Discomfort: Some people may have moderate gastrointestinal disturbances such as nausea, bloating, or abdominal pain.

2. Psychiatric Symptoms: Excessive or long-term usage of Mucuna Pruriens may cause psychiatric symptoms such as sleeplessness, anxiety, or disorientation.

3. Cardiovascular Effects: The presence of L-DOPA in Mucuna Pruriens may cause blood pressure changes, possibly impacting persons with cardiovascular disorders.

4. Allergic responses: Individuals who come into touch with the plant's surface may have allergic responses such as skin rashes or itching.

Drug Interactions

1. **MAO Inhibitors:** Mucuna Pruriens includes L-DOPA, which might cause hypertension when used with MAO inhibitors. Combining them should be avoided at all costs.

2. Mucuna Pruriens influences dopamine levels, therefore mixing it with dopamine antagonists used in antipsychotic drugs may reduce their efficacy.

3. **Antidiabetic medicines:** Because of the potential for additive effects on blood sugar levels, Mucuna Pruriens should be used with caution when used with antidiabetic medicines.

Contraindications And Precautions

1. **Pregnancy and nursing:** There is little information on its safety during pregnancy and nursing. As a result, it is advised to avoid using it during these times.

2. Individuals with mental problems, particularly psychosis or schizophrenia, should take Mucuna Pruriens with caution since it may increase symptoms.

3. Patients with kidney illness should see their doctor before taking Mucuna Pruriens since too much L-DOPA might impair renal function.

4. **Cardiovascular issues:** Those with heart diseases, high blood pressure, or other cardiovascular issues should exercise caution owing to the possibility of blood pressure changes.

While Mucuna Pruriens has a variety of medicinal properties, its usage requires careful evaluation and monitoring. Before using it, persons with pre-existing medical issues or those taking drugs should contact a healthcare expert to avoid any side effects or drug interactions. Monitoring for any unexpected symptoms or changes throughout its use is also recommended to guarantee its safe and efficient use.

CHAPTER 10

Future Perspectives

Emerging Trends In Mucuna Pruriens Research

The past decade has seen a spike in Mucuna Pruriens research, spurred by a rising interest in natural cures and traditional medicines. Several new trends have transformed the landscape of Mucuna Pruriens's research, indicating intriguing future paths for investigation.

• Precision medicine and personalized care:

• Advances in genetic research may open the road for individualized Mucuna Pruriens therapy. Understanding genetic variations and how they affect individual responses to Mucuna Pruriens compounds could lead to more targeted therapeutic interventions.

• **Combined Therapies:**

• Scientists are investigating the synergistic benefits of Mucuna Pruriens in combination with other herbal supplements or conventional pharmaceuticals. Combinatorial approaches have the potential to improve efficacy and address multifaceted health issues.

• **Increasing Bioavailability:**

• Research is being conducted to improve the bioavailability of active compounds in Mucuna Pruriens. New delivery systems and formulations may improve absorption, resulting in more consistent therapeutic results.

• **Environmental and Sustainability Concerns:**

• As people become more aware of the importance of sustainable practices, researchers are looking into eco-friendly cultivation methods for Mucuna Pruriens.

Mucuna Pruriens's research is increasingly incorporating sustainable sourcing and ethical harvesting practices.

Potential For Further Therapeutic Applications

• **Neurodegenerative Disorders Other Than Parkinson's:**

• While Mucuna Pruriens has shown promise in the treatment of Parkinson's disease, further research into its potential in other neurodegenerative disorders is ongoing. Mucuna pruriens may have therapeutic effects on Alzheimer's disease, Huntington's disease, and amyotrophic lateral sclerosis (ALS).

• **Psychiatric Disorders and Psychological Well-Being:**

• Mucuna Pruriens' effect on mental health extends beyond neurodegenerative conditions. Its potential for alleviating symptoms of anxiety, depression, and stress-related disorders is being investigated, as are its neuroprotective and mood-regulating properties.

• **Beyond Reproductive Health:**

• Mucuna Pruriens is being researched for broader reproductive health applications, in addition to its traditional use for enhancing fertility. Research into its effect on hormonal balance, menstrual irregularities, and conditions such as polycystic ovary syndrome (PCOS) is gaining traction.

• **Immunological and Metabolic Health:**

• Preliminary research suggests that Mucuna Pruriens could help with metabolic disorders and immune system modulation. Future research may reveal its role in diabetes, metabolic syndrome, and autoimmune disorders.

As we mark the first anniversary of our exploration of the multifaceted world of Mucuna Pruriens, it is clear that this botanical marvel has enormous therapeutic potential. Mucuna Pruriens' versatility is a testament to the richness of traditional medicinal knowledge, ranging from Parkinson's disease management to mental health benefits, sexual health, and beyond.

Emerging trends in Mucuna Prurien's research provide a glimpse of a future in which personalized, sustainable, and integrative healthcare approaches thrive. Collaboration between traditional wisdom and modern science becomes critical as we navigate this exciting terrain, fostering a holistic understanding of Mucuna Pruriens and its applications.

Finally, the adventure with Mucuna Pruriens has only just begun. The pages of research have yet to be written, and each discovery opens up new avenues for understanding and utilizing this botanical treasure's therapeutic potential. As we look forward to future discoveries, it is clear that Mucuna Pruriens will continue to captivate researchers, clinicians, and individuals looking for natural remedies for improved well-being.

Conclusion

Mucuna pruriens, also known as velvet bean or cowhage, is a leguminous plant that has gained popularity due to its diverse therapeutic properties. It's important to highlight key points about this remarkable plant as we dive into summarizing its significance and encouraging further exploration.

Summary Of Key Points Discussed

1. Mucuna pruriens contains bioactive compounds such as L-DOPA (levodopa), serotonin, and other alkaloids. L-DOPA, its main active ingredient, has been extensively researched for its neurological benefits, particularly in the treatment of Parkinson's disease symptoms.

2. Parkinson's Disease Management: Mucuna pruriens contains L-DOPA, making it a compelling natural alternative to synthetic L-DOPA in the treatment of Parkinson's disease. Studies have shown that it is effective in relieving motor symptoms while having fewer side effects than synthetic formulations.

3. Mucuna pruriens has shown promise in improving mood, reducing stress, and potentially aiding in depression and anxiety management, in addition to Parkinson's disease. It contains serotonin, which contributes to these mental health benefits.

4. Sexual Health and Fertility: The plant has been linked to increased male fertility due to its ability to increase testosterone levels and improve sperm quality. Anecdotal evidence suggests that it has aphrodisiac properties.

5. Other Therapeutic Uses: New research is looking into the plant's potential for diabetes management, weight management, and even antioxidant and anti-inflammatory properties.

Importance Of Mucuna Pruriens In Health And Medicine

Mucuna pruriens is significant because of its numerous health benefits. L-DOPA's natural occurrence is especially important in neurological conditions, providing a potential alternative to synthetic medications. Furthermore, its impact on mental health, sexual health, and potential applications in a variety of other conditions distinguishes it as a versatile botanical remedy.

Encouragement For Further Exploration And Utilization

While existing research provides promising results, there is still plenty of room for further investigation. Deeper research should be conducted in the following areas:

- **Optimized Formulations:** Creating standardized extracts or formulations to ensure consistent L-DOPA content and therapeutic effects.

- **Clinical Trials:** Large-scale, rigorous clinical trials to validate efficacy, safety, and appropriate dosage across diverse populations.

- **Understanding Mechanisms:** Investigating the mechanisms underlying its therapeutic actions to realize its full potential.

- **New Application Exploration:** Investigating its effects in conditions other than those currently being studied, such as neurodegenerative diseases other than Parkinson's, metabolic disorders, or even in skincare products for its antioxidant properties.

Finally, Mucuna pruriens is an intriguing natural resource with a variety of potential therapeutic benefits. Its role in the management of neurological, mental, and reproductive health issues, as well as its broader pharmacological actions, distinguishes it as a plant worthy of further scientific investigation and clinical validation. Its application could pave the way for novel treatments and interventions in a variety of medical domains, providing hope for improved health and well-being for people all over the world.

THE END

66